BODY BUILDING AFTER 40:

A COMPREHENSIVE GUIDE TO OPTIMAL NUTRITION FOR WOMEN

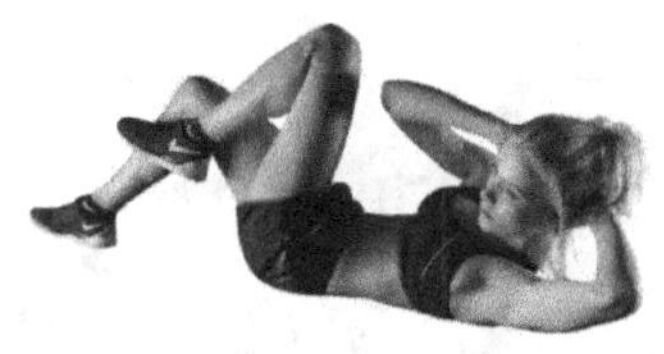

Unlock Your Potential and Transform

Your Body with a Targeted Diet Plan

Anna Moss

Copyright © 2023 by Anna Moss

All rights reserved

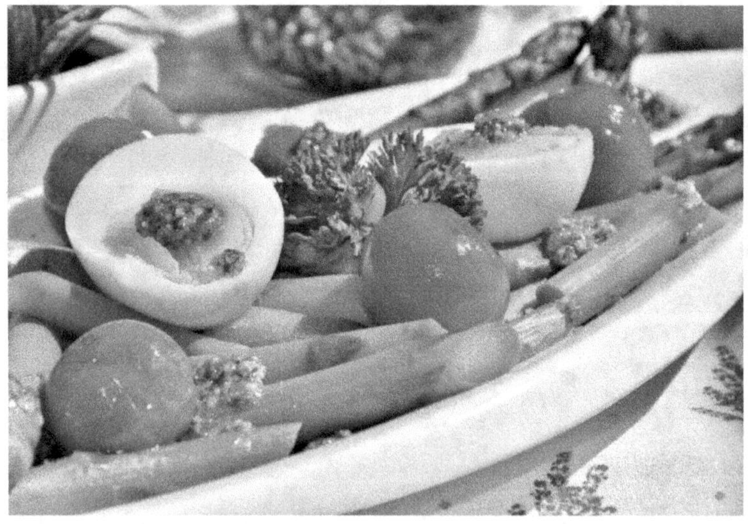

Table of Contents

INTRODUCTION

Viola had been a fitness enthusiast her whole life, but as she aged, she felt her body start to slow down. She was in her late 40s and she wanted to start bodybuilding, but she was worried that her age would hold her back.

Viola had heard about the benefits of bodybuilding, but she was concerned about how her body would react to the demands of an intense workout program. She decided to do some research and came across a book called "Body Building After 40: A Comprehensive Guide to Optimal Nutrition for Women."

Viola read the book from cover to cover and was surprised by how much information it provided. She learned about the importance of protein, carbohydrates, and fats in her diet, and how to properly structure her meals to maximize muscle growth. She also read about how to create an effective workout program that would help her reach her goals.

Viola followed the instructions in the book and her body responded positively. She was able to build lean muscle and lose fat while still maintaining her feminine shape. She was surprised at how quickly she was able to see results.

Viola felt more energized and confident than ever before. She was no longer worried about her age, but instead was proud that she was able to defy expectations and reach her goals. She had finally found a way to stay fit and healthy as she aged.

Viola was so pleased with the results she had achieved that she made it her mission to spread the word about bodybuilding after 40. She now actively coaches other women who are looking to take on this challenge, and she encourages them to read the same book that helped her reach her goals.

Bodybuilding is a form of strength training that is designed to increase muscle mass, strength, and overall physical health. It involves using resistance training, such as weightlifting, to build muscles and improve strength. Bodybuilding is a popular form of exercise, and it can be performed by people of all ages and fitness levels.

The introduction to bodybuilding is important for anyone interested in taking up the sport. It is important to understand the basic principles of bodybuilding so that you can develop a safe and effective workout routine. Before starting a bodybuilding program, it is important to consult with a qualified health care professional to make sure that it is right for you.

Once you have consulted with a health care professional and decided to start bodybuilding, it is important to understand the basics. You should develop a plan that includes a proper diet, rest, and exercise. The diet should be balanced, and should include plenty of protein, carbohydrates, and healthy fats. Rest is important to allow the body to recover and rebuild muscles. Exercise should involve resistance training, such as weightlifting, as well as cardiovascular exercise to help burn fat and improve overall fitness.

It is also important to understand the proper form for various exercises. Improper form can lead to injuries, so it is important to learn the correct way to perform each exercise.

Additionally, it is important to understand the importance of proper nutrition and supplementation. A good diet can help to fuel muscle growth, while supplementation can provide additional nutrients to support muscle growth.

Finally, it is important to understand the importance of motivation. Bodybuilding is a long-term commitment, and it is important to stay motivated to reach your goals. Staying motivated can involve varying your workouts, setting goals, and tracking your progress.

By understanding the basics of bodybuilding, you can ensure that you have the best possible experience. With a good plan and dedication, you can reach your bodybuilding goals.

CHAPTER 1:

Getting Started: The Basics of Bodybuilding

Many women become discouraged when they reach their 40s because they feel that they can't get the same results as younger women. However, that's simply not true. With the right approach, bodybuilding after 40 can be just as successful if not more than before.

The first step is to set realistic goals. It's important to understand that the body changes with age, and it won't respond to the same training program as it did when you were younger. Your expectations will need to be adjusted properly.

Next, you'll need to adjust your diet. As we age, our metabolism slows down and we may need to cut back on the number of calories we consume. Eating a balanced diet with lots of lean protein, healthy fats, and complex carbohydrates is essential for maintaining energy and muscle mass.

It's also important to ensure that you're getting enough rest. That means getting at least seven to eight hours of quality sleep every night. Sleep helps to restore energy and muscles, and it also helps with recovery after a workout.

Of course, you'll need to add an exercise program. Strength training is essential for building muscle and maintaining bone density. You can start with lighter weights and work your way up to heavier weights as you build strength and confidence. Also, it's important to add in some form of cardio activity to boost your metabolism and help with fat loss.

Finally, make sure that you're taking care of your body. That includes staying hydrated, stretching before and after workouts, and listening to your body. If you're feeling particularly sore or tired, it's okay to take a rest day.

Bodybuilding after 40 is absolutely possible for women. With patience, consistency, and the right approach, you can build the body you've always wanted.

What Is Bodybuilding?

Bodybuilding is an intense form of physical exercise that involves weight training, cardio and nutrition to build muscle, strength and endurance. Bodybuilding is a popular sport among men and women of all ages, but it can be especially beneficial for women over 40.

As women age, their bodies tend to lose muscle mass and bone mass, leading to a decrease in strength and an increase in body fat. Bodybuilding helps to counteract this natural process by encouraging the development of lean muscle mass and bone strength. This can help to improve posture, balance, and overall fitness levels.

Bodybuilding requires a commitment to regular workouts and a balanced diet that includes plenty of protein, healthy fats, and complex carbohydrates. It is important to choose exercises that target all major muscle groups, including the arms, chest, back, legs, and core. Exercises should be performed with the correct form and at a comfortable intensity level. Repetitions should be kept low and the weight should be adjusted to match the individual's strength level.

Nutrition is also an important factor in bodybuilding. Eating a balanced diet that is high in protein and healthy fats is essential for gaining muscle mass and losing fat. Eating several small meals throughout the day can help to ensure that the body has a steady supply of energy and nutrients to fuel workouts. Bodybuilding can be a great way for women over 40 to stay in shape and improve their overall health. It is important to consult with a doctor before beginning any bodybuilding program to ensure that it is safe and appropriate for the individual's age and fitness level. With the right approach and dedication, bodybuilding can be a great way to look and feel your best.

Benefits of Bodybuilding

Bodybuilding after 40 is becoming increasingly popular amongst women, and the benefits of this activity are numerous. Bodybuilding can help you maintain a healthy weight, increase your strength, improve your posture and flexibility, and even reduce the risk of certain diseases and health conditions.

Here are some of the key benefits of bodybuilding

1. A faster metabolism, which is the body's mechanism for either burning body fat for energy or storing it as fat. With the appropriate exercise, you can change your body's chemistry such that fat continues to burn long after the exercise session has ended.

2. Improves the strength, rigidity, and tone of our muscles, which improves both our appearance and our ability to perform. Even the padding out of our skin to remove wrinkles is aided by firmer, more toned muscles.

3. Improving and repairing bone strength and density – strong bones help prevent and treat osteoporosis. Walking, a low-intensity activity, is insufficient to activate the connected muscles and stress the bones; only strength training will accomplish this.

4. Increases our body's endurance, energy, and stamina, enabling us to complete our daily tasks with ease and yet have energy left over to engage in enjoyable activities.

5. Strong leg muscles and our abdominal muscles stabilize us, lowering our chance of falling and improving balance. When we fall, our bones and joints are protected by our powerful muscles, which act as cushions.

6. Lower chance of disease: A strong immune system goes hand in hand with a strong overall body. The immune system draws upon the proteins that are stored in muscle tissue as necessary. In particular, the "big three" of diabetes, cancer, and heart disease, a stronger immune system lowers the chance of illness.

7. More lean muscle mass is your buddy because it will assist you either shed more weight or control your weight. The daily calorie expenditure increases by 35–50 for every additional pound of muscle. You wouldn't even be able to tell if you put on a few extra pounds of lean muscle, but you would see how much thinner and trimmer you would seem.

8. Injury Prevention – A strong foundation fortifies our tendons, ligaments, and bones. By gradually increasing your strength around the affected area, you can use strength training to recuperate and assist with rehabilitation after an injury.

9. Better athletic, exercise, and everyday performance, such as carrying children or shopping or climbing stairs. Being more physically healthy and strong makes everything we do simpler and more fun.

10. Better mental health - When you improve your physical health through appropriate exercise, you'll be more alert, focused, and able to concentrate better. You'll also experience less anxiety and depression and an uptick in general mood and attitude.

11. Aging is easier since a strong physique is built with strong muscles. For the purpose of fending off the consequences of aging, a strong body also has a strong mind. Aging bodies remain functional with the help of strength training and fitness.

Strength training helps us feel good, gain confidence, and maintain a healthy self-esteem. It also tones our muscles, which improves how we appear and makes us feel better about ourselves. To live our lives to their fullest potential, these things are crucial.

Understanding Your Baseline

Understanding your baseline is an important part of any bodybuilding program, especially for women over 40. It's the starting point for knowing where you are and how far you need to go to reach your goals. Knowing your baseline helps you to set realistic goals for yourself and to track your progress over time.

Your baseline is the amount of physical activity and strength you have when you begin a bodybuilding program. This includes your body composition, strength level, and cardiovascular fitness. Your body composition is the percentage of fat and muscle in your body.

Knowing your body fat percentage can be helpful in setting realistic goals. Your strength level is the amount of weight you can lift and the number of repetitions you can do.

Lastly, your cardiovascular fitness is the level of your aerobic endurance and ability to complete activities like running or cycling.

When it comes to bodybuilding, you want to make sure that your baseline is as accurate as possible. Taking the time to measure your body composition, strength, and cardiovascular fitness will help you set realistic goals and track your progress over time.

You can use a variety of tools to measure your baseline, including fitness trackers, body fat calipers, and fitness tests. You can also consult with a personal trainer or nutritionist to get a more accurate assessment.

By understanding your baseline, you can set realistic goals and create a bodybuilding program that works for you. You can then track your progress over time to ensure that you are reaching your goals. This will help you stay motivated to keep going and make progress. When it comes to bodybuilding for women over 40, understanding your baseline is key to success.

Creating an effective workout program

Nutrition and exercise are important components of a body building program, especially for those over 40. Women over 40 should focus on building a program that is tailored to their specific needs and goals.

First and foremost, an effective workout program should include strength training. Strength training is essential for maintaining muscle strength and mass as we age. Women should focus on compound movements such as squats, deadlifts, and overhead presses. These exercises target multiple muscles and joints which helps to build strength and muscles.

Second, cardiovascular exercise should be included in the program. Cardiovascular exercise, such as running, cycling, and swimming, can help to improve aerobic capacity and burn calories. This type of exercise is important for improving heart health and overall fitness.

Third, flexibility and mobility exercises should be included in the program. These exercises help to increase flexibility and reduce the risk of injury. Stretching and yoga are great choices for increasing flexibility and mobility.

Finally, nutrition should also be a part of the program. Eating a balanced diet that includes plenty of fruits, vegetables, lean proteins, and healthy fats is essential for reaching body building goals.

Supplements can also be beneficial for women over 40 to ensure they are getting the necessary nutrients to support their body building program.

In conclusion, creating an effective workout program in relation to body building after 40 is essential for women to maintain their health and fitness. Strength training, cardiovascular exercise, flexibility and mobility exercises, and nutrition should all be included in the program. By following this program, women over 40 can build muscle and strength, improve aerobic capacity, maintain flexibility, and improve their overall nutrition.

CHAPTER 2

Nutrition for Bodybuilding

When it comes to bodybuilding for women over 40, nutrition is essential for achieving and maintaining the body of your dreams. Nutrition for bodybuilding is all about creating an environment that optimizes muscle growth and fat loss. It's important to understand that bodybuilding is a lifestyle and that nutrition plays a major role in achieving your goals.

The first step to proper nutrition for bodybuilding is to determine your body's caloric needs. A calorie is a unit of energy and the body requires certain amounts of energy in order to function optimally. Knowing your caloric needs allows you to plan your meals accordingly and maintain a balance between calorie intake and calorie expenditure.

Once you've determined your body's caloric needs, the next step is to ensure you're getting the right types of foods. Bodybuilding nutrition is all about consuming the right types of macronutrients in the right proportions. Macronutrients are carbohydrates, proteins, and fats.

Each of these macronutrients has a specific role in the bodybuilding process and should be consumed in the right amounts.

Carbohydrates are the body's main source of energy and should be the main source of calories for bodybuilding. Carbohydrates should be mainly complex carbohydrates such as whole grains, oats, brown rice, quinoa, and sweet potatoes. Simple carbohydrates such as white bread, white rice, and sugary snacks should be consumed in moderation.

Protein is the building block of muscle and is essential for muscle growth. Protein should be consumed throughout the day in small amounts and should come from lean sources such as lean beef, poultry, fish, and eggs. Protein shakes are also a great way to increase your daily protein intake.

Fats are essential for proper hormone production and should be consumed in moderate amounts. Healthy fats such as avocados, olive oil, nuts, and seeds are great sources of essential fatty acids.

In addition to macronutrients, micronutrients such as vitamins, minerals, and antioxidants are also essential for optimal health and bodybuilding. Eating a variety of fruits, vegetables, and other plant-based foods is the best way to ensure you're getting all the essential micronutrients.

Finally, when it comes to bodybuilding nutrition for women over 40, it's important to remember to drink plenty of water. Water helps to keep your body hydrated and aids in the digestion and absorption of nutrients. Aim for 8 to 10 glasses of water per day.

By following these nutrition guidelines for bodybuilding, you can be sure that you're creating an environment for optimal muscle growth and fat loss. Nutrition is an essential part of bodybuilding and should not be overlooked. With proper nutrition and a solid training program, you can achieve the body of your dreams.

The Role of Protein

Women lose muscular mass as they get older, and their body composition changes. Goals for bodybuilding may become more difficult as a result, especially beyond age 40. Protein is crucial for maintaining and growing muscles, and it can play a significant role in a bodybuilding regimen for women over 40.

A macronutrient called protein is made up of amino acids. These amino acids support the growth and repair of the body's tissues, including muscle tissue. Due to hormonal changes, decreased physical activity, and other causes, women are more prone to develop muscle loss as they age. Consuming adequate protein might assist prevent this muscle loss and make it simpler to achieve bodybuilding objectives.

Protein can help women over 40 feel filled for longer periods of time, which can help them stick to their diet plan and help them build and retain muscle. Increased protein intake can also aid in lowering cravings for harmful foods. Women who are trying to lose weight may find this to be extremely helpful.

Any bodybuilding regimen must include protein, and women over 40 should try to consume 1.2–1.7 grams of protein per kilogram of body weight per day. Eating a range of foods, such as lean meats, fish, eggs, dairy, nuts and seeds, legumes, and soy products, will help you achieve this. To meet daily protein targets, protein shakes and other supplements can be beneficial.

Women over 40 who want to grow muscle can still succeed by including protein in their diets. A diet that includes enough protein can help people lose weight, control cravings, and build and retain muscle. To get the most out of protein for bodybuilding, women should try to consume 1.2–1.7 grams of protein per kilogram of body weight per day.

Macro-nutrients and Calories

Beyond age 40, bodybuilding for women can be a great way to keep active and in shape, but it's crucial to understand the macronutrients and calorie requirements for this. The primary nutrients in diet, such as proteins, carbs, and fats, are known as macronutrients. They each give the body energy and play a unique part in metabolism and wellness.

The energy needed for bodybuilding comes from calories, so it's critical to consume enough of them to power your workouts.

There are three macro nutrients protein, carbohydrates and fats:

Protein

When it comes to constructing lean muscle mass, protein reigns first among the macronutrients. Your body can only employ one of the three, and that is the one, to develop new muscle.

You should therefore consume a lot of it by eating high-quality foods.

Fish, poultry, eggs, red meat, milk, and whey are the finest foods for high protein content. If you want to see the biggest muscle gains, consume a lot of these meals. Consume at least one of these, or better yet, a combination of them, with every meal. Each pound of body weight, try to consume at least one gram of protein.

Carbohydrates

Energy, minerals, and fiber are all abundant in carbohydrates. Just fruits and vegetables should be consumed if you want to gain lean muscular mass. They provide very high concentrations of the vitamins and minerals you require to build muscle mass and foster an anabolic environment.

In terms of calorie and nutritious content per weight, all other carbohydrates fall short of fruits and vegetables. They will provide you with the greatest fiber to aid in the digestion of all the protein you will be consuming daily.

Fats

Your primary energy source will be fats. They have a well-known reputation for significantly raising testosterone levels by up to 300%. Avocados, olive oil, butter, cream, coconut cream, almonds, almond butter, egg yolks, and meat and poultry fats are examples of healthy fats that you should consume. The greatest way to grow muscle is to consume mostly saturated and monounsaturated fats. Avoid trans fatty acids and exercise caution while consuming polyunsaturated fats because they can become unstable.

The fact that fats provide 9 calories per gram, compared to the other two macronutrients' 4 calories per gram, makes them a significant source of energy. They also don't create an insulin spike, so your body can keep burning fat all day long.

Your body requires calories as fuel to power workouts and daily tasks. To maintain their busy lifestyles, women over 40 should try to consume at least 1,200 calories daily. Your activity level will determine the precise number of calories you should consume, therefore it is advisable to speak with a dietitian or nutritionist to get an accurate figure.

Micro-nutrients

Women over 40 who are interested in bodybuilding can benefit immensely from taking a closer look at their micro-nutrient intake. Micro-nutrients are essential vitamins and minerals needed for optimal health. These nutrients help with muscle repair and growth, hormone balance, energy production and immune system support.

Vitamin B1 (Thiamin). Meats, whole grains, fruit, nuts, fortified breakfast cereals, and veggies all contain this. Thiamin, a kind of vitamin B1, is crucial because it facilitates the release of energy from carbs. Moreover, it must actively interact with the heart and neurological system. A human body will therefore be unable to function properly and fulfil its obligations without this nutrient. The body will experience undesirable effects as a result of the unleashed energy from the carbohydrates.

Vitamin B2 (Riboflavin). Green vegetables, mushrooms, fortified morning cereals, legumes, liver, milk, rice, and eggs are all good sources of this vitamin. Its primary duty is to discharge energy derived from macronutrients like glucose, protein, and fat.

It also participates in the metabolism and transportation of iron. The regular structure and operations of the skin and bodily linings are likewise under its control.

Vitamin B3 (Niacin). Consuming foods like wheat, maize, eggs, meat, dairy products, and yeast is a natural way to get this nutrient. For a healthy neurological system, brain function, and production of sex hormones, vitamin B3 is essential. Its functions and health advantages include helping the body cleanse or eliminate pollutants that would otherwise be harmful. A healthy digestive system and production of healthy skins are beneficial. Moreover, vitamin B3 can lower cholesterol and high blood pressure while improving blood circulation.

Vitamin B6 (Pyridoxine). Brewer's yeast, oats, wheat, sardines, beef, mackerel, free-range eggs, poultry, bananas, avocados, cabbage, brown rice, dried fruit, and molasses are good sources of vitamin B6. The immune system is strengthened by vitamin B6, which also eases cramps, nausea, and vomiting. It has anti-aging ingredients and is best for treating skin and nervous system issues.

Moreover, this vitamin defends against cancer's ad hoc onslaught. The body won't be able to absorb enough vitamin B12 if vitamin B6 isn't consumed.

Vitamin B12 (Cobalamin) The following foods should be consumed to obtain this vitamin: Liver, Cheese, Free Range Eggs, Kidney, Beef, Oily Fish, Milk, Fortified Cereals, Lamb, and Pork. Vitamin B12 is responsible for producing red blood cells and maintaining the health of the nervous system. It is one of the most crucial B-group vitamins, to the point where staunch vegetarians are advised to take doses of this vitamin. Its range of capabilities includes preventing anaemia, boosting energy, being a healthy component for growth, and stimulating hunger, particularly in children. It is also important for maintaining a healthy neurological system and for improving cognitive functions.

Folic acid and foliate. Liver, peanuts, almonds, citrus fruits, carrots, green leafy vegetables, apricots, cantaloupe melons, avocados, beans, beetroot, broccoli, free range eggs, and liver are all excellent sources of folic acid. It is a component of the vitamin B complex and one among the vitamins whose intake is most overlooked.

Vitamin C Blackcurrants, broccoli, green peppers, kiwi fruits, Brussels sprouts, lemons, oranges, strawberries, cabbage, and any other types of fruits with the same or similar components from the fruits containing Vitamin C mentioned are good food sources for vitamin C. and other veggies that are rich in vitamin C. This vitamin is crucial for keeping bodily tissues organized and functioning regularly as well as acting as an antioxidant, which stops the body from being harmed. It significantly increases the body's ability to absorb iron from non-meat sources. Also, it aids in the process of healing any wounds brought on by physical harm of any kind.

Other Considerations

Bodybuilding for women after 40 is a great way to stay fit, healthy, and motivated. It can also help to improve self-confidence and create a sense of accomplishment. However, there are a few other considerations that should be taken into account when engaging in bodybuilding after 40.

First, bodybuilding after 40 can be more strenuous than bodybuilding in younger years. As the body ages, it naturally loses muscle mass, making it more difficult to build and maintain muscle. Therefore, it is important to start at a lower intensity and gradually work up to a higher intensity as the body adjusts and becomes stronger.

Second, women after 40 should consider the health risks associated with bodybuilding. While bodybuilding can be beneficial for overall health, it can also cause strain on the joints and muscles, leading to injury. Therefore, it is important to speak with a doctor or physical therapist before beginning a bodybuilding regimen to ensure the body is healthy enough for the activity.

Third, it is important to create a plan for bodybuilding that fits into a woman's lifestyle. This may include creating a schedule for workouts, as well as setting realistic goals that can be achieved over time. Additionally, it is important to ensure that there is enough time for rest and recovery between workouts.

Fourth, women after 40 should consider the cost of bodybuilding. Although there are many free resources available, such as bodyweight exercises, some equipment may need to be purchased. Additionally, supplements may need to be purchased to aid in muscle building and recovery.

In conclusion, bodybuilding for women after 40 can be a great way to stay fit, healthy, and motivated. However, there are several other considerations that should be taken into account when engaging in bodybuilding after 40, such as health risks, lifestyle, and cost. By taking these considerations into account, women can create a safe and effective bodybuilding plan that works for them.

CHAPTER 3

Meal Planning for Bodybuilding

Meal planning for bodybuilding can be a daunting task for any bodybuilder, but especially so for women over 40. Bodybuilding is an effective way to get in shape and build muscle, but it also requires a specific approach to nutrition. Meal planning is an important part of any bodybuilding program, and it is even more important for women over 40 who are bodybuilding.

First and foremost, it is important to understand that the bodybuilding diet for women over 40 needs to be tailored to meet their individual needs. As women age, their bodies change, and their nutritional needs may be different than those of a younger bodybuilder. Additionally, women over 40 may have different goals than younger bodybuilders, such as maintaining a healthy weight and preventing age-related muscle loss.

When it comes to meal planning for bodybuilding, it is important to focus on quality over quantity. Women over 40 should focus on eating quality proteins, complex carbohydrates, healthy fats, and plenty of fruits and vegetables. It is also important to ensure that the meals are balanced and provide adequate calories and nutrients to support muscle growth and performance.

In addition to focusing on quality nutrition, women over 40 also need to focus on portion control. Eating too much at each meal can lead to weight gain and interfere with muscle growth. As a result, it is important to measure and weigh food to ensure accurate portion sizes.

Finally, it is important to make sure that the meal plan is varied and interesting. Boredom with meal planning can lead to overeating and unhealthy food choices. It is important to try new recipes, switch up ingredients, and make meals fun and exciting.

Meal planning for bodybuilding can be a daunting task, but with a little planning and preparation, it is possible for women over 40 to create a meal plan that meets their individual needs and supports their bodybuilding goals. With the right approach to nutrition and meal planning, women over 40 can achieve their bodybuilding goals and maintain a healthy lifestyle.

Day 1

Breakfast:

Omelette with spinach, mushrooms and feta cheese

Snack:

Greek yogurt and mixed berries and nuts

Lunch:

Grilled salmon with quinoa, grilled vegetables

Snack: Protein shake with banana

Dinner:

Roasted turkey breast with mashed sweet potatoes and
steamed green beans

Day 2

Breakfast:

High-fiber cereal with low-fat milk and banana

Snack:

Hummus with cucumber and carrots

Lunch:

Baked chicken with brown rice and steamed broccoli

Snack:

Greek yogurt with mixed berries and nuts

Dinner:

Grilled tuna with quinoa, grilled vegetables

Day 3

Breakfast:

Smoothie with Greek yogurt, berries and chia seeds

Snack:

Hard-boiled egg with sliced tomato

Lunch:

Grilled Portobello mushroom burger with sweet potato fries

Snack:

Protein shake with banana

Dinner:

Baked cod with brown rice and steamed vegetables

Day 4

Breakfast:

Oatmeal with apples, walnuts and cinnamon

Snack:

Apple slices with peanut butter

Lunch:

Grilled shrimp with quinoa, grilled vegetables

Snack:

Greek yogurt with mixed berries and nuts

Dinner:

Baked salmon with mashed sweet potatoes and steamed green beans

Day 5

Breakfast:

Egg white omelette with spinach, tomatoes and feta cheese

Snack:

Hummus with cucumber and carrots

Lunch: G

rilled chicken with quinoa, grilled vegetables

Snack:

Protein shake with banana

Dinner:

Baked cod with mashed sweet potatoes and steamed green beans

Day 6

Breakfast:

Avocado toast with poached egg

Snack:

Greek yogurt with mixed berries and nuts

Lunch:

Grilled turkey burger with sweet potato fries

Snack:

Hard-boiled egg with sliced tomato

Dinner:

Grilled salmon with brown rice and steamed broccoli

Day 7

Breakfast:

Smoothie with Greek yogurt, berries and chia seeds

Snack:

Apple slices with peanut butter

Lunch:

Baked chicken with quinoa, grilled vegetables

Snack:

Protein shake with banana

Dinner:

Grilled tuna with mashed sweet potatoes and steamed green beans

Setting Goals

At any age, setting goals for bodybuilding is crucial to your fitness journey's success. Yet, the objectives you establish for bodybuilding should be specific to your needs. According to research, older women can benefit from strength training, but they may need to adapt their objectives to account for the physical changes brought on by aging. Here are some pointers for making bodybuilding goals beyond 40 that are reasonable and doable.

Start by making a reasonable evaluation. It's crucial to evaluate your present fitness level and take an honest look in the mirror before making any bodybuilding goals. In what areas are you strong and weak? How much have you already accomplished? Setting more attainable goals will be easier if you make a realistic appraisal of your current capabilities.

Choose an objective that is doable. Make sure your bodybuilding goals are attainable and reasonable when you establish them for yourself. While pushing oneself is a wonderful thing, it's also crucial to set goals you can actually accomplish in the allotted time.

Make both immediate and long-term goals. You can stay motivated and monitor your progress by setting both short-term and long-term goals. Short-term objectives may include things like gaining strength or enhancing your form when performing specific workouts. Long-term objectives can be more challenging, like competing in a bodybuilding contest or losing a certain amount of weight.

Don't be too hard on yourself. Being patient with oneself is one of the most crucial things to keep in mind while setting bodybuilding goals after 40. It's acceptable if you don't get results right away. You will eventually accomplish your goals if you are persistent and dedicated.

Be aware of your body. Your body may change as you get older, so you might need to modify your expectations and goals accordingly. Pay attention to your body and what it is trying to tell you. Don't push yourself too hard or ignore any red flags if anything doesn't feel right.

Keep your eye on your objectives. It can be challenging to set objectives for bodybuilding beyond 40, but it's crucial to remain motivated and focused.

Keep a progress log, acknowledge your accomplishments, and don't let failures demoralize you. Your bodybuilding objectives are attainable with commitment and effort.

Calculating Macros

It can seem intimidating to calculate macros for bodybuilding for women over 40, but it doesn't have to be. Our bodies don't respond to exercise the same way they did when we were younger as we age because our metabolism slows down. In order to take the right actions to achieve our fitness goals, it is crucial to understand the body's unique needs.

Identifying your daily calorie needs is the first step in calculating macros for bodybuilding for women over 40. You can do this by utilizing an online calculator that takes your age, sex, height, weight, and degree of activity into account. The next step is to calculate your macro-nutrient requirements after determining your daily caloric needs.

Protein is crucial for bodybuilding since it aids in muscle growth and repair. Protein consumption for women over 40 should range from 1.2 to 1.7 g/kg of lean body mass. A calculator online can also be used to figure this out.

Carbohydrates are crucial for bodybuilding since they give you the energy you need to execute. For women over 40, the Recommended Dietary Allowance (RDA) for carbs is 130–230 g/day. It's crucial to remember that these are only suggestions and that everyone has different needs.

Additionally necessary for muscle growth, fats should not account for more than 30% of your daily caloric intake. Hormone production, energy production, and cell function all depend on healthy fats like those found in nuts, avocados, and olive oil.

You may develop the ideal food plan for your bodybuilding goals once you've identified your daily caloric needs, your macro needs, and your fat needs. It's critical to keep in mind that each person has unique nutritional requirements and that there is no one-size-fits-all strategy.

A nutritionist or dietitian should be consulted if you are unsure of your macro-nutrient requirements.

A crucial step in accomplishing your fitness objectives is figuring out your macro-nutrient requirements for bodybuilding for women over 40. With the correct knowledge and advice, you can develop the perfect meal plan to help you attain your goals.

CHAPTER 4

Supplements for Bodybuilding

Bodybuilding for women over 40 can be intimidating. After all, your body is changing and you may not be as strong as you once were. But you can still take steps to stay fit and healthy, and one way to do that is to add supplements to your diet. Supplements for bodybuilding are formulated to maximize the benefits of exercise and help you reach your goals.

Protein is essential for muscle growth and repair. Adding a protein supplement to your diet can help you get the necessary nutrients to fuel your body and get the most out of your workouts. Look for a supplement that contains whey, casein, and egg protein, as these are all high-quality sources of protein.

Creatine is another supplement that can help with bodybuilding. It helps to increase muscle size and strength, and has been shown to be especially beneficial for women. It can help you achieve your goals faster, and can also make workouts more effective.

Beta-alanine is another supplement that can help with bodybuilding. This amino acid helps to increase endurance and strength, and can also delay muscle fatigue. This allows you to push yourself further in your workouts and get the most out of them.

Omega-3 fatty acids are important for overall health, but they are especially beneficial for bodybuilding. They can help reduce inflammation, which can help you recover faster from workouts and reduce the risk of injury. They can also help boost your metabolism and improve your overall energy levels.

These are just some of the supplements that can help with bodybuilding. Be sure to talk to your doctor before taking any supplements, as they can interact with certain medications and could cause adverse reactions. It's also important to choose a supplement that is specifically formulated for bodybuilding, as they are specifically designed to meet the needs of older adults. With the right supplement, you can reach your bodybuilding goals and stay fit and healthy.

Protein Powders

Bodybuilding for women over 40 is a popular and increasingly mainstream form of exercise. One of the key components of any bodybuilding routine is protein supplementation. Protein powders are a convenient and efficient way to supplement your protein intake, and can be tailored to meet the specific needs of bodybuilders over 40.

Protein is an essential macronutrient that makes up the building blocks of muscle tissue. As women over 40 are at a higher risk of muscle loss, the importance of adequate protein intake is paramount. Protein powders provide a convenient and cost-effective way to supplement your protein intake and can help to maximize muscle growth.

When selecting a protein powder for bodybuilding, it is important to consider the type of protein, the amino acid profile and the added ingredients. Generally, whey protein is the most popular choice, as it is a complete protein source with an excellent amino acid profile. Other popular options include soyo milk, egg, and casein proteins.

It is also important to consider the added ingredients, as some protein powders can contain high amounts of added sugar, artificial sweeteners and other additives.

Women over 40 may also benefit from specialized protein blends that are specifically tailored for bodybuilding. These protein powders may contain higher amounts of leucine, an essential amino acid that is involved in muscle protein synthesis. Additionally, some blends may contain added ingredients such as creatine and BCAAs that may help to further enhance muscle growth.

When supplementing with protein powder, it is important to remember that diet and exercise are still the most important components of any bodybuilding routine. Protein powder should be used to supplement your protein intake and should never be used as a meal replacement. Additionally, it is important to consult with a health professional before beginning any new supplement routine.

In conclusion, protein powders are a convenient and cost-effective way to supplement your protein intake and can help to maximize muscle growth for bodybuilders over 40.

When selecting a protein powder, it is important to consider the type of protein, the amino acid profile and the added ingredients. Additionally, specialized protein blends may be beneficial for bodybuilding. Remember that diet and exercise are still the most important components of any bodybuilding routine, and protein powder should be used to supplement your protein intake and not as a meal replacement.

Pre-Workout Supplements

Pre-workout supplements are gaining popularity amongst bodybuilders of all ages, especially women over 40. As women age, their energy levels, strength, and muscle mass tend to decline. Pre-workout supplements can help to combat this decline by increasing energy and endurance, improving muscle size and strength, and helping to promote recovery from workouts.

Pre-workout supplements are designed to provide a boost of energy and focus before a workout. They typically contain a combination of ingredients such as caffeine, B vitamins, and amino acids, which can increase energy levels and mental focus. They can also contain ingredients such as creatine, beta-alanine, and citrulline malate, which can help improve muscle size, strength, and endurance.

Women over 40 may benefit from pre-workout supplements because they are more likely to experience fatigue and decreased motivation during their workouts. By providing a boost of energy and focus, pre-workout supplements can help them to stay motivated and push through their workouts. Additionally, the ingredients in pre-workout supplements can help to increase muscle size, strength, and endurance, which can be beneficial for bodybuilders of any age.

It's important to note that pre-workout supplements should be used in moderation and should not be used as a substitute for a healthy diet and regular exercise.

They should be taken as recommended on the label and should be avoided by those who have any pre-existing medical conditions. Additionally, they should not be taken in combination with other stimulants or supplements without consulting a doctor first.

Overall, pre-workout supplements can be a great addition to a bodybuilding regimen for women over 40. They can provide a boost of energy and focus and can help to improve muscle size, strength, and endurance. Be sure to read the labels carefully and talk to your doctor about any potential risks before taking pre-workout supplements.

Post-Workout Supplements

Post-workout supplements for women over 40 are an important part of any bodybuilding program. As we age, our bodies become less efficient at utilizing the nutrients from our food. This can lead to a decrease in muscle mass, strength, and overall health. Post-workout supplements provide the essential nutrients needed to support the body's recovery and rebuilding process. They can also help to reduce soreness, improve joint health, and increase energy levels.

The most important post-workout supplement for women over 40 is protein. Protein helps to rebuild and repair muscle tissue and also helps to reduce muscle breakdown. Women over 40 should aim to consume around 20-30 grams of protein within 30 minutes of exercise. Good sources of protein include whey, casein, and plant-based proteins.

Creatine is also an important post-workout supplement for women over 40. Creatine aids in boosting muscular mass and power.Moreover, it enhances recuperation and lessens weariness.. Women should aim to consume around 5-10 grams of creatine daily.

BCAAs are also important for post-workout recovery in women over 40. BCAAs help to reduce muscle soreness, improve muscle growth, and reduce fatigue. Women should aim to consume around 5-10 grams of BCAAs post-workout.

Glutamine is another post-workout supplement that can be beneficial to women over 40. Glutamine helps to reduce muscle breakdown, improve muscle growth, and reduce fatigue. Women should aim to consume around 5-10 grams of glutamine post-workout.

Finally, a post-workout multivitamin and mineral supplement can be beneficial. These supplements help to replenish nutrients that may have been lost during exercise. They can also help to improve energy levels and overall health.

In conclusion, post-workout supplements can be an important part of any bodybuilding program for women over 40. They help to replenish lost nutrients, reduce muscle breakdown, and improve overall health. Consuming protein, creatine, BCAAs, glutamine, and a multivitamin and mineral supplement post-workout can help to maximize recovery and results.

Other Supplements

Bodybuilding is a great way to stay fit and healthy. However, while strength training and diet are essential components of a successful bodybuilding routine, taking the right supplements can help make the process easier.

The most common supplements used by bodybuilders are protein, creatine, and amino acids. Protein is essential for muscle growth and repair and is best taken before and after workouts.

Creatine helps to increase the body's energy levels during workouts and is usually taken in the morning.

Amino acids help to build muscle and reduce muscle breakdown and can be taken before or after workouts.

Other supplements that may be beneficial for bodybuilding for women over 40 include omega-3 fatty acids, which can help to reduce inflammation and support overall health. Additionally, branch-chain amino acids can help to promote muscle growth and reduce muscle breakdown.

Multivitamins can also be beneficial for bodybuilders, as they provide important vitamins and minerals that can help to support overall health and wellness. Additionally, probiotics can help to support digestive health and boost the immune system.

if you're interested in taking supplements for bodybuilding, it's important to speak to your doctor first. They can help you determine which supplements are best for your body and lifestyle. Additionally, it's important to stick to the recommended dosage for each supplement and use them in conjunction with a healthy diet and exercise routine.

By taking the right supplements, bodybuilders over 40 can get the most out of their workouts and help to reach their bodybuilding goals. With the right combination of strength training, diet, and supplements, bodybuilding over 40 can be a great way to stay fit and healthy.

CHAPTER 5:

Putting It All Together

Bodybuilding for women over 40 can seem like a daunting task. After all, it's not the same as it was when you were younger. The good news is that with the right approach, you can still reach your goals.

Putting it all together when it comes to bodybuilding for women over 40 means focusing on the basics. You'll need to pay attention to your diet, your workout routine, and your recovery. All of these elements will help you to maximize your results.

When it comes to your diet, you'll want to focus on eating a balanced diet that is low in processed foods and high in lean proteins, healthy fats, and complex carbohydrates. This will ensure that you are getting the proper nutrients to help you reach your goals. You'll also want to make sure that you're snacking on healthy foods throughout the day to keep your energy levels up.

Your workout routine should be tailored to your goals. If you are looking to build muscle, you'll want to focus on compound movements like squats, deadlifts, and presses. If you are looking to lose fat, you'll want to focus on more cardio-based exercises like running, cycling, and swimming.

Finally, you'll need to make sure that you are taking the time to recover. This means taking days off after a hard workout and getting plenty of sleep each night. You'll also want to make sure that you are taking time to stretch and foam roll to help you stay limber and prevent injury.

Putting it all together when it comes to bodybuilding for women over 40 means focusing on the basics. Pay attention to your diet, your workout routine, and your recovery. This will help you to reach your goals and make sure that you stay healthy and fit.

Exercise Program

Exercise programs for bodybuilding in women over 40 are becoming increasingly popular. As women age, their bodies change and it is important to adjust their exercise routine to meet their changing needs. Bodybuilding for women over 40 requires a combination of strength training and cardio workouts to achieve optimal results.

Strength training is essential for developing muscle mass, which helps to boost the metabolism and burn fat. Moreover, it aids in increasing bone density and lowering the risk of osteoporosis. The American College of Sports Medicine recommends that women over 40 strength train two to three times per week. Exercises should target all the major muscle groups of the arms, legs, back, chest, and abdominals. For best results, use a combination of free weights and machines.

Cardio exercises are important for improving cardiovascular health and burning calories. Women over 40 should aim for at least 30 minutes of moderate-intensity cardio exercises such as walking, jogging, cycling, or swimming at least three times per week.

High-intensity interval training (HIIT) is also beneficial for burning fat and increasing endurance.

Nutrition is another important factor for bodybuilding in women over 40. Eating a balanced diet that is rich in lean proteins, healthy fats, and complex carbohydrates is essential for building muscle and keeping the body healthy. Consuming adequate amounts of protein is particularly important for preserving muscle mass while dieting.

Finally, it is important to stay motivated and consistent with your exercise program. Setting realistic goals and tracking progress can help to keep you encouraged and motivated. Additionally, working with a personal trainer or joining a fitness class can help to keep you accountable and make your workouts more enjoyable.

By following a personalized exercise program that combines strength training and cardio workouts with a healthy diet, women over 40 can successfully build muscle and reach their bodybuilding goals.

Personalised exercise program

1. Lower body resistance training:

a. Squats (body weight, barbell, or dumbbells)

b. Lunges (body weight, barbell, or dumbbells)

c. Step-ups (body weight, barbell, or dumbbells)

d. Deadlifts (body weight, barbell, or dumbbells)

e. Glute bridges (body weight, barbell, or dumbbells)

f. Leg presses (machine or body weight)

g. Leg extensions (machine)

h. Leg curls (machine)

2. Upper body resistance training:

a. Chest presses (barbell, dumbbells, or machine)

b. Push-ups (body weight)

c. Shoulder presses (barbell, dumbbells, or machine)

d. Bent-over rows (barbell, dumbbells, or machine)

e. Lat pull-downs (machine)

f. Bicep curls (barbell, dumbbells, or machine)

g. Tricep extensions (barbell, dumbbells, or machine)

3. Core training:

a. Planks

b. Side planks

c. Bridge

d. Bicycle crunches

e. Russian twists

4. Cardio:

a. Walking

b. Jogging

c. Swimming

d. Cycling

e. Elliptical

f. Rowing

5. Stretching:

a. Dynamic stretching

b. Static stretching

c. Yoga

d. Pilates

e. Foam rolling

6. Recovery:

a. Massage

b. Ice baths

c. Contrast baths

d. Epsom salt baths

e. Sauna

f. Sleep

Nutrition Program

Women over 40 have unique nutritional needs when it comes to bodybuilding. They require a balanced diet that provides all the essential nutrients to build muscle and stay healthy. A nutrition program for bodybuilding should include an emphasis on consuming quality proteins, healthy fats, and complex carbohydrates. It should also include adequate hydration and regular meals to keep energy levels up.

Protein is essential for muscle building. Women over 40 should consume 1.5-2.0 grams of protein per pound of body weight per day. Quality proteins sources include lean meats, poultry, fish, eggs, nuts, legumes, and dairy products. Make an effort to include them in each meal.

Fats provide energy and help absorb essential vitamins and minerals. Eating healthy fats, such as olive oil, avocados, and nuts, can help support muscle growth. Consume about 20-30% of your daily calories from healthy fats.

Carbohydrates are important for providing energy and fuel for workouts. Complex carbohydrates, such as whole grains, fruits, and vegetables, are the best choice. Aim to consume 3-4 servings of complex carbohydrates per day.

Hydration is also important for bodybuilding. Drinking plenty of water throughout the day will help keep your body hydrated and your muscles functioning.

In addition to a balanced diet, regular meals are important for bodybuilding for women over 40. Eating smaller meals throughout the day can help keep your energy levels up and your metabolism running. Eating a variety of foods from all the food groups will provide the essential nutrients you need for bodybuilding.

To ensure optimal results, it's important to consult a registered dietitian or nutritionist to create an individualized nutrition program for bodybuilding. They will be able to tailor a plan to meet your individual needs and help you reach your goals.

Recovery and Injury Prevention

Bodybuilding can be a great way to stay in shape and build strength, but it's important to be aware of the risks of injury and the importance of proper recovery and injury prevention for women over 40 who are bodybuilding. As we get older, our bodies become more susceptible to injury, so it's important to take the necessary precautions to keep yourself safe while still achieving your fitness goals.

Here are some tips on recovery and injury prevention:

1. Warm Up and Cool Down – Warming up and cooling down are essential for any type of physical activity, but it's especially important for bodybuilding women over 40. A warm up helps to increase blood flow to the muscles, increase flexibility, and reduce the risk of injury. Cooling down is also important for reducing the risk of injury and allowing the body to recover.

2. Listen to Your Body – It's important to listen to your body and take rest days as needed. When your body is tired or sore, it's important to take a break and allow your muscles to recover before jumping back into bodybuilding.

Ignoring the signs of fatigue or soreness can increase the risk of injury.

3. Don't Push Too Hard – It's important to challenge yourself with bodybuilding, but it's also important to make sure you're not pushing yourself too hard. Over-exerting yourself can lead to injury, so it's important to listen to your body and stay within your limits.

4. Don't Forget to Stretch – Stretching before and after bodybuilding is important for increasing flexibility and reducing the risk of injury. It's also important to stretch after each exercise to help the muscles recover.

5. Use Proper Form – Proper form is essential for avoiding injury while bodybuilding. Make sure you're using the correct form for each exercise, and consult with a trainer or coach if you're unsure.

6. Take Breaks – Taking breaks between sets and exercises can help the body recover and reduce the risk of injury. Make sure to rest for at least 30 seconds between sets, and take a few minutes break between exercises.

7. Drink Plenty of Water – Staying hydrated is essential for recovery and injury prevention. Make sure to drink plenty of water before, during, and after your bodybuilding session to replenish any fluids lost through sweating.

By following these tips, bodybuilding women over 40 can stay safe and reduce the risk of injury while still achieving their fitness goals. Remember to listen to your body, take breaks, use proper form, and stretch before and after bodybuilding to ensure a safe and successful workout.

BONUS

Delicious recipes for bodybuilders

1. Chicken and Spinach Salad:

Ingredients:

- 2 cups of cooked chicken, diced

- 2 cups of fresh spinach, chopped

- 1/2 cup of cherry tomatoes, diced

- 1/4 cup of red onion, diced

- 1/4 cup of feta cheese, crumbled

- 2 tablespoons of olive oil

- 1 tablespoon of apple cider vinegar

- 1/2 teaspoon of sea salt

- 1/4 teaspoon of black pepper

Instructions:

1. In a large bowl, combine the cooked chicken, spinach, tomatoes, red onion and feta cheese.

2. In a separate bowl, whisk together the olive oil, apple cider vinegar, salt and pepper.

3. Pour the dressing over the salad and toss to combine.

4. Serve chilled or at room temperature.

2. Lentil and Kale Stir Fry:

Ingredients:

- 1 cup of dry lentils, cooked

- 2 tablespoons of olive oil

- 1 onion, diced

- 2 cloves of garlic, minced

- 1 red bell pepper, diced

- 4 cups of kale, chopped

- 1/2 teaspoon of sea salt

- 1/4 teaspoon of black pepper

Instructions:

1. Heat the olive oil in a large skillet over medium heat.

2. Add the onion and garlic and cook until fragrant, about 2 minutes.

3. Add the bell pepper and cook for an additional 2 minutes.

4. Add the cooked lentils, kale, salt and pepper.

5. Cook, stirring occasionally, until the kale is wilted and the lentils are heated through, about 5 minutes.

6. Serve warm.

3. Baked Salmon with Basil Pesto:

Ingredients:

- 2 salmon fillets

- 1 tablespoon of olive oil

- 1/4 teaspoon of sea salt

- 1/4 teaspoon of black pepper

- 1/4 cup of basil pesto

Instructions:

1. Preheat oven to 400°F.

2. Place the salmon fillets on a baking sheet lined with parchment paper.

3. Drizzle with olive oil and season with salt and pepper.

4. Bake for 15 minutes or until the salmon is cooked through.

5. Remove from the oven and top with basil pesto.

6. Serve warm.

4. Quinoa Edamame Bowl:

Ingredients:

- 1 cup of quinoa, cooked

- 1 cup of edamame, cooked

- 1 red bell pepper, diced

- 1/4 cup of red onion, diced

- 2 tablespoons of olive oil

- 1 tablespoon of apple cider vinegar

- 1/4 teaspoon of sea salt

- 1/4 teaspoon of black pepper

Instructions:

1. In a large bowl, combine the cooked quinoa, edamame, bell pepper and red onion.

2. In a separate bowl, whisk together the olive oil, apple cider vinegar, salt and pepper.

3. Pour the dressing over the quinoa mixture and toss to combine.

4. Serve chilled or at room temperature.

5. Zucchini Noodle Salad:

Ingredients:

- 2 large zucchini, spiralized

- 1 red bell pepper, diced

- 1/2 cup of cherry tomatoes, diced

- 1/4 cup of red onion, diced

- 2 tablespoons of olive oil

- 1 tablespoon of balsamic vinegar

- 1/4 teaspoon of sea salt

- 1/4 teaspoon of black pepper

Instructions:

1. In a large bowl, combine the zucchini noodles, bell pepper, tomatoes and red onion.

2. In a separate bowl, whisk together the olive oil, balsamic vinegar, salt and pepper.

3. Pour the dressing over the salad and toss to combine.

4. Serve chilled or at room temperature.

6. Greek Yogurt Parfait:

Ingredients:

- 2 cups of plain Greek yogurt

- 1/2 cup of fresh berries

- 1/4 cup of nuts, chopped

- 1/4 cup of granola

Instructions:

1. In a large bowl, combine the yogurt and berries.

2. Layer the yogurt mixture and nuts in a parfait glass.

3. Top with granola and serve.

7. Tuna Avocado Wrap:

Ingredients:

- 2 whole wheat wraps

- 2 cans of tuna, drained and flaked

- 1 avocado, mashed

- 1/4 cup of red onion, diced

- 2 tablespoons of olive oil

- 1 tablespoon of lemon juice

- 1/4 teaspoon of sea salt

- 1/4 teaspoon of black pepper

Instructions:

1. Place the wraps on a clean work surface.

2. In a small bowl, combine the tuna, avocado, red onion, olive oil, lemon juice, salt and pepper.

3. Spread the tuna mixture onto the wraps.

4. Roll up the wraps and cut in half.

5. Serve chilled or at room temperature.

8. Sweet Potato Hash:

Ingredients:

- 2 large sweet potatoes, peeled and diced

- 1 red bell pepper, diced

- 1/2 cup of mushrooms, diced

- 1/4 cup of red onion, diced

- 2 tablespoons of olive oil

- 1/2 teaspoon of sea salt

- 1/4 teaspoon of black pepper

Instructions:

1. Heat the olive oil in a large skillet over medium heat.

2. Add the sweet potatoes, bell pepper, mushrooms and red onion.

3. Cook, stirring occasionally, until the sweet potatoes are golden and cooked through, about 10 minutes.

4. Season with salt and pepper.

5. Serve warm.

9. Veggie Burger:

Ingredients:

- 1/2 cup of cooked quinoa

- 1/2 cup of cooked black beans

- 1/4 cup of oats

- 1/4 cup of walnuts, chopped

- 1/4 cup of carrots, grated

- 1/4 cup of red onion, diced

- 1/4 teaspoon of sea salt

- 1/4 teaspoon of black pepper

Instructions:

1. In a food processor, combine the quinoa, black beans, oats, walnuts, carrots, red onion, salt and pepper.

2. Process until everything is combined and the mixture is slightly sticky.

3. Form the mixture into 4 patties.

4. Heat a large skillet over medium heat.

5. Add the veggie burgers and cook until golden and cooked through, about 5 minutes per side.

6. Serve warm.

10. Broccoli and Cheese Frittata:

Ingredients:

- 8 eggs

- 1/4 cup of milk

- 1/2 teaspoon of sea salt

- 1/4 teaspoon of black pepper

- 1 tablespoon of olive oil

- 1/2 cup of broccoli, chopped

- 1/4 cup of red onion, diced

- 1/2 cup of cheddar cheese, shredded

Instructions:

1. Preheat oven to 375°F.

2. In a large bowl, whisk together the eggs, milk, salt and pepper.

3. Heat the olive oil in an oven-safe skillet over medium heat.

4. Add the broccoli and onion and cook until softened, about 5 minutes.

5. Pour the egg mixture into the skillet.

6. Sprinkle with cheese and cook until the edges are set, about 5 minutes.

7. Transfer to the oven and bake until the center is set, about 10 minutes.

8. Serve warm.

11. Baked Apple Cinnamon Oatmeal:

Ingredients:

- 2 cups of rolled oats

- 1 teaspoon of ground cinnamon

- 1/4 teaspoon of sea salt

- 1/4 cup of brown sugar

- 2 apples, peeled and diced

- 1/2 cup of milk

- 1/4 cup of walnuts, chopped

- 2 tablespoons of butter, melted

Instructions:

1. Preheat oven to 375°F.

2. In a large bowl, combine the oats, cinnamon, salt, brown sugar and apples.

3. In a separate bowl, whisk together the milk, walnuts and butter.

4. Pour the milk mixture into the oats mixture and stir to combine.

5. Pour the oatmeal mixture into a greased baking dish.

6. Bake for 30 minutes or until the top is golden brown.

7. Serve warm.

12. Coconut Quinoa Porridge:

Ingredients:

- 1 cup of quinoa, cooked

- 2 cups of coconut milk

- 1/4 teaspoon of sea salt

- 1 banana, mashed

- 1/4 cup of shredded coconut

- 2 tablespoons of honey

Instructions:

1. In a medium saucepan, combine the cooked quinoa, coconut milk and salt.

2. Bring to a boil, reduce heat to low, cover and simmer for 15 minutes.

3. Remove from heat and stir in the mashed banana, shredded coconut and honey.

4. Serve warm.

13. Baked Sweet Potato Fries:

Ingredients:

- 2 large sweet potatoes, peeled and cut into wedges

- 2 tablespoons of olive oil

- 1/2 teaspoon of sea salt

- 1/4 teaspoon of black pepper

Instructions:

1. Preheat oven to 425°F.

2. Place the sweet potato wedges on a baking sheet lined with parchment paper.

3. Drizzle with olive oil and season with salt and pepper.

4. Bake for 25 minutes or until golden and crisp.

5. Serve warm.

14. Avocado Toast:

Ingredients:

- 2 slices of whole wheat bread

- 1 avocado, mashed

- 1/4 teaspoon of sea salt

- 1/4 teaspoon of black pepper

Instructions:

1. Toast the bread until golden.

2. Spread the mashed avocado onto the toast.

3. Sprinkle with salt and pepper.

4. Serve warm.

15. Lentil Soup:

Ingredients:

- 1 tablespoon of olive oil

- 1 onion, diced

- 2 cloves of garlic, minced

- 2 carrots, diced

- 2 celery stalks, diced

- 1 can of diced tomatoes

- 1 cup of dry lentils, rinsed

- 6 cups of vegetable broth

- 1/2 teaspoon of sea salt

- 1/4 teaspoon of black pepper

Instructions:

1. Heat the olive oil in a large pot over medium heat.

2. Add the onion and garlic and cook until fragrant, about 2 minutes.

3. Add the carrots, celery, tomatoes, lentils, vegetable broth, salt and pepper.

4. Bring to a boil, reduce heat to low and simmer for 25 minutes or until the lentils are tender.

5. Serve warm.

16. Roasted Vegetable Salad:

Ingredients:

- 2 cups of broccoli, chopped

- 2 cups of cauliflower, chopped

- 1 cup of cherry tomatoes, halved

- 1/4 cup of red onion, diced

- 2 tablespoons of olive oil

- 1 tablespoon of balsamic vinegar

- 1/4 teaspoon of sea salt

- 1/4 teaspoon of black pepper

Instructions:

1. Preheat oven to 400°F.

2. Place the broccoli, cauliflower, tomatoes and onion on a baking sheet lined with parchment paper.

3. Drizzle with olive oil and season with salt and pepper.

4. Roast for 20 minutes or until golden and tender.

5. In a large bowl, whisk together the balsamic vinegar, salt and pepper.

6. Pour the dressing over the roasted vegetables and toss to combine.

7. Serve chilled or at room temperature.

17. Greek Salad with Chickpeas:

Ingredients:

- 2 cups of romaine lettuce, chopped

- 1/2 cup of cucumber, diced

- 1/2 cup of cherry tomatoes, halved

- 1/4 cup of feta cheese, crumbled

- 1/2 cup of cooked chickpeas

- 2 tablespoons of olive oil

- 1 tablespoon of lemon juice

- 1/4 teaspoon of sea salt

- 1/4 teaspoon of black pepper

Instructions:

1. In a large bowl, combine the lettuce, cucumber, tomatoes, feta cheese and chickpeas.

2. In a separate bowl, whisk together the olive oil, lemon juice, salt and pepper.

3. Pour the dressing over the salad and toss to combine.

4. Serve chilled or at room temperature.

18. Baked Banana Oatmeal:

Ingredients:

- 2 cups of rolled oats

- 1/4 teaspoon of sea salt

- 1 teaspoon of ground cinnamon

- 2 bananas, mashed

- 1/2 cup of milk

- 1/4 cup of walnuts, chopped

- 2 tablespoons of butter, melted

Instructions:

1. Preheat oven to 375°F.

2. In a large bowl, combine the oats, salt, cinnamon, mashed bananas, milk, walnuts and butter.

3. Pour the oatmeal mixture into a greased baking dish.

4. Bake for 30 minutes or until the top is golden brown.

5. Serve warm.

19. Quinoa and Kale Stuffed Peppers:

Ingredients:

- 2 large bell peppers, halved and seeded

- 1 cup of quinoa, cooked

- 2 cups of kale, chopped

- 1/4 cup of red onion, diced

- 1/4 cup of feta cheese, crumbled

- 2 tablespoons of olive oil

- 1 tablespoon of balsamic vinegar

- 1/4 teaspoon of sea salt

- 1/4 teaspoon of black pepper

Instructions:

1. Preheat oven to 375°F.

2. Place the bell pepper halves in a greased baking dish.

3. In a large bowl, combine the cooked quinoa, kale, red onion and feta cheese.

4. In a separate bowl, whisk together the olive oil, balsamic vinegar, salt and pepper.

5. Pour the dressing over the quinoa mixture and toss to combine.

6. Stuff the bell peppers with the quinoa mixture.

7. Bake for 25 minutes or until the peppers are tender.

8. Serve warm.

20. Baked Cod with Spinach:

Ingredients:

- 2 cod fillets

- 2 tablespoons of olive oil

- 1/4 teaspoon of sea salt

- 1/4 teaspoon of black pepper

- 2 cups of spinach

- 1/4 cup of cherry tomatoes, halved

- 2 cloves of garlic, minced

Instructions:

1. Preheat oven to 400°F.

2. Place the cod fillets on a baking sheet lined with parchment paper.

3. Drizzle with olive oil and season with salt and pepper.

4. Bake for 15 minutes or until the cod is cooked through.

5. Heat the remaining olive oil in a large skillet over medium heat.

6. Add the spinach, tomatoes and garlic and cook until wilted, about 5 minutes.

7. Serve the cod with the spinach mixture.

Smoothie recipes

1. Blueberry-Banana Smoothie:

Ingredients:

1 banana,

1/2 cup frozen blueberries,

1/2 cup plain Greek yogurt,

1/4 cup almond milk,

1 teaspoon honey

Preparation and Instruction:

1. Add all the ingredients to a blender and blend until smooth.

2. Drink 1-2 times per day as part of your bodybuilding regime.

2. Strawberry-Mango Smoothie:

Ingredients:

1 cup frozen strawberries,

1/2 cup frozen mango,

1/2 cup plain Greek yogurt,

1/4 cup almond milk,

1 teaspoon honey

Preparation and Instruction:

1. Add all the ingredients to a blender and blend until smooth.

2. Drink 1-2 times per day as part of your bodybuilding regime.

3. Avocado-Banana Smoothie:

Ingredients:

1 banana,

1/2 avocado,

1/2 cup plain Greek yogurt,

1/4 cup almond milk,

1 teaspoon honey

Preparation and Instruction:

1. Add all the ingredients to a blender and blend until smooth.

2. Drink 1-2 times per day as part of your bodybuilding regime.

4. Pineapple-Banana Smoothie:

Ingredients:

1 banana,

1/2 cup frozen pineapple,

1/2 cup plain Greek yogurt,

1/4 cup almond milk,

1 teaspoon honey

Preparation and Instruction:

1. Add all the ingredients to a blender and blend until smooth.

2. Drink 1-2 times per day as part of your bodybuilding regime.

5. Peanut Butter-Banana Smoothie:

Ingredients:

1 banana,

2 tablespoons peanut butter,

1/2 cup plain Greek yogurt,

1/4 cup almond milk,

1 teaspoon honey

Preparation and Instruction:

1. Add all the ingredients to a blender and blend until smooth.

2. Drink 1-2 times per day as part of your bodybuilding regime.

6. Coconut-Mango Smoothie:

Ingredients:

1/2 cup frozen mango,

1/2 cup coconut milk,

1/2 cup plain Greek yogurt,

1/4 cup almond milk,

1 teaspoon honey

Preparation and Instruction:

1. Add all the ingredients to a blender and blend until smooth.

2. Drink 1-2 times per day as part of your bodybuilding regime.

7. Strawberry-Banana-Ginger Smoothie:

Ingredients:

1 banana,

1/2 cup frozen strawberries,

1 teaspoon fresh ginger,

1/2 cup plain Greek yogurt,

1/4 cup almond milk,

1 teaspoon honey

Preparation and Instruction:

1. Add all the ingredients to a blender and blend until smooth.

2. Drink 1-2 times per day as part of your bodybuilding regime.

8. Acai-Blueberry Smoothie:

Ingredients:

1/2 cup frozen blueberries,

1/2 cup frozen acai berries,

1/2 cup plain Greek yogurt,

1/4 cup almond milk,

1 teaspoon honey

Preparation and Instruction:

1. Add all the ingredients to a blender and blend until smooth.

2. Drink 1-2 times per day as part of your bodybuilding regime.

9. Raspberry-Banana Smoothie:

Ingredients:

1 banana,

1/2 cup frozen raspberries,

1/2 cup plain Greek yogurt,

1/4 cup almond milk,

1 teaspoon honey

Preparation and Instruction:

1. Add all the ingredients to a blender and blend until smooth.

2. Drink 1-2 times per day as part of your bodybuilding regime.

10. Kale-Banana Smoothie:

Ingredients:

1 banana,

1 cup kale,

1/2 cup plain Greek yogurt,

1/4 cup almond milk,

1 teaspoon honey

Preparation and Instruction:

1. Add all the ingredients to a blender and blend until smooth.

2. Drink 1-2 times per day as part of your bodybuilding regime.

11. Green Apple-Cucumber Smoothie:

Ingredients:

1/2 cucumber,

1/2 green apple,

1/2 cup plain Greek yogurt,

1/4 cup almond milk,

1 teaspoon honey

Preparation and Instruction:

1. Add all the ingredients to a blender and blend until smooth.

2. Drink 1-2 times per day as part of your bodybuilding regime.

12. Carrot-Orange Smoothie:

Ingredients:

2 carrots,

1 orange,

1/2 cup plain Greek yogurt,

1/4 cup almond milk,

1 teaspoon honey

Preparation and Instruction:

1. Add all the ingredients to a blender and blend until smooth.

2. Drink 1-2 times per day as part of your bodybuilding regime.

13. Mango-Papaya Smoothie:

Ingredients:

1/2 cup frozen mango,

1/2 cup frozen papaya,

1/2 cup plain Greek yogurt,

1/4 cup almond milk,

1 teaspoon honey

Preparation and Instruction:

1. Add all the ingredients to a blender and blend until smooth.

2. Drink 1-2 times per day as part of your bodybuilding regime.

14. Coconut-Banana Smoothie:

Ingredients:

1 banana,

1/2 cup coconut milk,

1/2 cup plain Greek yogurt,

1/4 cup almond milk,

1 teaspoon honey

Preparation and Instruction:

1. Add all the ingredients to a blender and blend until smooth.

2. Drink 1-2 times per day as part of your bodybuilding regime.

15. Pear-Cinnamon Smoothie:

Ingredients:

1 pear,

1 teaspoon ground cinnamon,

1/2 cup plain Greek yogurt,

1/4 cup almond milk,

1 teaspoon honey

Preparation and Instruction:

1. Add all the ingredients to a blender and blend until smooth.

2. Drink 1-2 times per day as part of your bodybuilding regime.

16. Peach-Banana Smoothie:

Ingredients:

1 banana,

1/2 cup frozen peaches,

1/2 cup plain Greek yogurt,

1/4 cup almond milk,

1 teaspoon honey

Preparation and Instruction:

1. Add all the ingredients to a blender and blend until smooth.

2. Drink 1-2 times per day as part of your bodybuilding regime.

17. Carrot-Ginger Smoothie:

Ingredients:

2 carrots,

1 teaspoon fresh ginger,

1/2 cup plain Greek yogurt,

1/4 cup almond milk,

1 teaspoon honey

Preparation and Instruction:

1. Add all the ingredients to a blender and blend until smooth.

2. Drink 1-2 times per day as part of your bodybuilding regime.

18. Spinach-Banana Smoothie:

Ingredients:

1 banana,

1 cup spinach,

1/2 cup plain Greek yogurt,

1/4 cup almond milk,

1 teaspoon honey

Preparation and Instruction:

1. Add all the ingredients to a blender and blend until smooth.

2. Drink 1-2 times per day as part of your bodybuilding regime.

19. Avocado-Mango Smoothie:

Ingredients:

1/2 avocado,

1/2 cup frozen mango,

1/2 cup plain Greek yogurt,

1/4 cup almond milk,

1 teaspoon honey

Preparation and Instruction:

1. Add all the ingredients to a blender and blend until smooth.

2. Drink 1-2 times per day as part of your bodybuilding regime.

20. Coconut-Pineapple Smoothie:

Ingredients:

1/2 cup frozen pineapple,

1/2 cup coconut milk,

1/2 cup plain Greek yogurt,

1/4 cup almond milk,

1 teaspoon honey

Preparation and Instruction:

1. Add all the ingredients to a blender and blend until smooth.

2. Drink 1-2 times per day as part of your bodybuilding regime.

CONCLUSION

Bodybuilding for women after 40 is a safe and effective activity that can promote physical and mental health. It can help to reduce the risks associated with age-related health issues, such as obesity and low bone density, as well as providing an enjoyable, low-impact form of exercise. Additionally, it can be a great way for women over 40 to stay active, gain confidence, and improve their overall quality of life. Ultimately, it is important to consult with a medical professional before embarking on any exercise program, particularly when it comes to bodybuilding, to ensure that the activity is safe and appropriate for the individual's age and health status.

Overall, bodybuilding is a safe and rewarding activity that can help women over 40 stay healthy and active. As long as it is done with caution and proper guidance, it can be a great way to stay in shape and improve overall health.

www.ingramcontent.com/pod-product-compliance
Lightning Source LLC
Chambersburg PA
CBHW070846250726
48662CB00003B/1383